Healthy Life Food

If you must leave a healthy life watch your intake

Isah Abdulwali Garba

ISBN: 9798387154249

DEDICATION

This book is dedicated to my parents Mr./Mrs. Garba Omeji and to my friends and relations and to those who have not found my contents yet.

CONTENTS

Introduction

In basic terms the body has two altogether different and complex frameworks of fuel delivering sources. As energy is imperative to the actual presence of human action and endurance the two-energy style rely upon one another for help. This book shows you what food varieties give you the most energy. It happens so regularly - we resolve to happen with a wellbeing and actual work out regime with zing and probable much exhibition as well; in any case, in the principal seven day stretch of going into the arrangement, all that dwindles. Can anyone explain why we don't stay with the eating routine plans, the early daytime running plans, the actual activity designs that we make? Furthermore, how may we guarantee we continue onward with these plans, for the good of our own and for the people that are reliant upon us? Is it safe to say that you are eating just to fulfill your craving or to make your taste buds cheerful? Or then again would you say you are eating to assume better control over your life? In this digital book, we perceive how you can make your life substantially more ideal essentially by causing a direct that you eat accurately.

THE Essentials

Energy is required for the different capabilities like support of development, everyday exercises, practice and numerous different developments or capabilities that are frequently underestimated. These are divided among the two energy frameworks. In this day and age, only here and there do any wellbeing and wellness plans work. What is the justification behind their disturbing pace of disappointment? The world is much less refreshing than it was twenty years prior. Much of this is ascribed to the modified food propensities for people. The Rudiments The essential and first to be utilized energy framework is the high-impact framework. This framework involves oxygen for the capability of the muscles and requests a considerable amount from the general body framework. This request generally builds the rate and profundity of breathing and blood supply primarily on account of the relating increment of the pulse. At the point when the body requires more energy, which can't be met because of the raised requirement for more oxygen than the body framework consequently changed to the anaerobic energy framework. This framework can create energy without the need to utilize oxygen. This energy is produced through the reasonable or right utilization of food sources. The food varieties devoured direct the sorts of energy levels everybody can create. Muscle weariness as a rule happens when all the energy sources are depleted which can be credited to various reasons; the most convincing one relies particularly upon the kinds of food varieties eaten. There are a few classes of food sources that produce different valuable components for the human body framework and taking note of the ones that make or upgrade the energy creating sources is helpful to be aware of. Hence, this information ought to assist the person with picking the right kinds of food sources. The high-impact framework works by separating the sugars, unsaturated fats and amino acids in the food varieties eaten while the anaerobic framework sets energy free from the food sources put away in the body, generally during extreme action sessions. In the event that we catch wind of the disappointment of diets or exercise center plans surrounding us, normally it isn't their issue. Usually, the shortcoming of the people began with much upheaval about going through these plans, enlightening every one of their associates and collaborators, and afterward didn't submit to those projects. The people who leave the activity or count calories midway don't see the benefits, normally, and everyone faults the arrangement. What the world needs these days is certainly not a new wellbeing or work out regime or an eating routine, yet it requires inspiration. It needs the right kind of mentality to completely finish any plan they have decided as far as possible. In the event that they can do that, the greater part of the medical problems that are connected with way of life circumstances will become old fashioned. Furthermore, we don't need to visit the sides of the earth to find this inspiration. The inspiration lies here, inside us; we essentially have to look through it out and use it. One age back, people wouldn't fantasize about getting anything low quality food they might set up to take care of their appearances. These days, that's what we do so nonchalantly. "I'm ravenous" usually signifies "I need a burger or a sausage, probably with chips as an afterthought and some cola." And, "I'm on a tight eating routine" signifies "I'm on a synthetically ridden pill which will overcome my yearning and deny my collection of nutrients." It's truly no big surprise that we are confronting so many medical problems today. Our wellbeing is a mark of what we consume. The sorry condition that we're living in is certainly not a singular issue; it's a worldwide issue. The world is eating inaccurately. Six in ten people in the US are overweight, and the number will be eight in each ten people when we hit 2021. Might it be said that we are genuinely contemplating this? We aren't. Indeed, even as you're concentrating on this digital book, you probably have a parcel of chips as an afterthought. Do you have any idea that what you spent on that bundle, which is filling your stomach with the absolute most harmful synthetic substances known to mankind, would rather have taken care of a gaunt young person in Rwanda? However, it's not just about being magnanimous. It's about ourselves as well. Indeed, we must be childish. With such horrifying wellbeing figures, would we confirm or deny that we are setting out toward destruction? We're certainly not eating right. Whatever abundance stuff that brings - corpulence and the different medical afflictions afterward - we must be ready for it. So, the following time you see that a program has fizzled or is getting a great deal of analysis, recall that the analysis isn't most likely in light of the fact that the program remains in dangerous territory. Much of the time, it is on the grounds that individuals started with incredible goals and afterward didn't follow the program as they ought to have.

THE Manner in which YOU Ponder FOOD

The most vital thing that you want to keep your wellbeing and work out regime alive - significantly more urgent than an educator or a specialist - is your own intention. You are not entirely set in stone to examine what is going on. In this way, you're overweight and are pushing off a couple of pounds. No rec center educator from wherever on the planet will help you on the off chance that you don't go to sufficient lengths to have the right eating regimen and to adhere to your standard activity. Regardless of whether you're debilitated and are taking a gander at treatment, no doctor will help in the event that is not entirely set in stone in following the treatment stage, whether it's taking the drug at the right time or swearing off certain food sources. Your Mentality We have wandered horrendously with our dietary patterns so far. Assume control won't improve. The number 1 thing is mindfulness. We need to realize what food varieties are right for ourselves and what are not. We need to return to preparing and understand what the supplements are that your body genuinely needs and in what sum. Then we need to fabricate a dietary routine for us as well as our friends and family so we eat better. We need to eliminate every one of the food sources that are antagonistic - the sugars, the fats, the starches, we don't genuinely need them - and integrate food sources that might support our wellbeing. This sounds excessively sermonizing, I get it. However, that is the main relief we have. Assuming we keep crunching on Oreos, we're never going to improve. Be that as it may, there's trust. Trust lies in the way that there are a ton of food varieties out there that are basically essentially as delicious as those terrible low-quality foods yet we have hardly any familiarity with them. These are the food varieties that we have barely any familiarity with yet, we probably could do without them or as we don't have the foggiest idea how to fix them, yet a solid cookbook might help you in grasping grouped fascinating ways to sound cooking. Indeed, even with a similar kind of diet you eat, you can invoke a few truly flavorful sound dishes. Indeed, it's all a lot of conceivable. You can change your dietary patterns to a major degree, while simultaneously taking care of your sense of taste. The truth of the matter is that the weight reduction industry is capable in a critical manner towards this defeat of the created human race. They show us captivating before-after photos of an individual with a foot-long sub and afterward the very fellow with 6 pack abs and let us know that the eating routine made that conceivable. In any case, the truth of the matter is, if we somehow happened to get our heads together, we may handily do that as well, without burning through 1000s of dollars on those eating regimens. Also, what do we need to do? 2 general things: - Control what we consume. Enjoy actual effort. Presently, is that a lot to achieve? Don't we owe that to our body that has served us so well for such an extremely long time? Don't we owe that to ourselves and our friends and family?

HONEY AND Entire GRAINS

Throughout the long-term honey has been demonstrated to the one supporting power behind the energy circle. Helping the human body in different regions it is first still unmatched in its energy delivering element. Honey is nature's most normal energy promoter. It likewise goes about as a powerful invulnerability framework developer while giving the normal solution for a large group of different illnesses as well. Energy is vital to the smooth streaming normal of an everyday existence pattern of any person. Hence, finding energy sources that are both steady and solid are critical to staying in shape and blissful. A Decent Pair The regular advantages of honey have been generally recognized and acknowledged. Other than its extraordinary taste, honey is likewise a characteristic wellspring of sugar, which is an energy creator for helping execution, perseverance and decreasing degrees of muscle exhaustion. This is particularly helpful for competitors. The sugar content in the honey assists with assuming a part in forestalling exhaustion during exercise meetings and furthermore during instructional meetings for sports devotees. These sugars are separated into glucose and fructose and capabilities in various however praising ways. The glucose content in the honey is by and large consumed at a quicker rate and emits a prompt jolt of energy while the fructose works at a slower speed for a more maintainable and delayed energy dispensing. With regards to tending to glucose levels in the body framework, honey has been known to assist with keeping the levels steady. As honey is a wonderful food item and it's normal in its structure, eating it's anything but an undeniably challenging activity. Individuals of any age are for the most part very ready to consume honey in any of its ways. It's even well-known with kids. The energy created from consuming a limited quantity of honey everyday assists youngsters with adapting to the actual kinds of day-to-day school exercises and sports responsibilities. For the grown-ups too, consuming an everyday little portion of honey can go quite far in keeping the energy levels at its best during a requesting day at work. Making sandwiches with honey with different fillings is one approach to making a wonderful tidbit. Applying honey on a newly toasted cut of bread is likewise a welcome breakfast elective. Adding honey to drinks as opposed to utilizing sugar is supported. The vast majority today need a handy solution for their energy helping necessities and this normally comes in the unfortunate types of sports beverages, espresso and refined starches like sugar and keeping in mind that bread. However, these produce the ideal increased energy levels, it ought to be noticed that this energy is genuinely brief and the sleepiness that follows is normally more intensely felt. Thus, picking to consume some type of entire grains isn't just a superior other option but at the same time is a lot better. Entire grains give the energy that arrives in a more mind-boggling structure that separates over a more extended timeframe. This then makes the stage for supporting the energy levels for longer periods. In light of its more complicated make up the entire grains accompany a variety of valuable components like minerals, nutrients, phytonutrients, and fiber which are additionally wealthy in fiber. Adding the entire grain fixings is any dish frequently finishes the flavor or upgrades it by and large. Entire grains can have different structures like wheat, oat, grain, maize, earthy colored rice, faro, spelt, emmer, einkorn, rye, millet, buckwheat, and some more. These can then be made into different items like entire wheat flour, entire wheat bread, entire wheat pasta, moved oats or oat groats, triticale flour, popcorn and teff flour. The advantages of consuming entire grains reliably can assist with diminishing the gamble of coronary illness, lower cholesterol levels safeguard against many sorts of malignant growth and aid weight the board. Entire grains ought not be mistaken for its lesser and more refined "cousin". However refined grains have a few advantages. It is in every case better to settle in general grain options.

NUTS AND LEAN MEAT

Nuts are a significant wellspring of supplements for both human and creature utilization. Being wealthy in an entire host of essential supplements it very well may be eaten in its crude structure, cooked or as an added substance to currently previous dishes. Though nuts are characterized as a hard-shelled organic product, there are numerous different food varieties that are remembered for the nut family. Various sorts of meats for the most part add to different flavors; but the best kind is the one with however much lean meat content as could reasonably be expected. Its undisputed truth is that the meats that contain a lot of fat are a culinary treat to be sure yet for wellbeing purposes finding an opportunity to comprehend the advantages of consuming lean meats is extremely quite insightful. Great Proteins And Oils It is currently considered normal information that nuts enormously help in holding a ton of diseases under control or from happening by any means. For example, nuts have been known to have the option to keep the chance of coronary heart sickness showing, in any event, for those entirely coming from a long queue of relatives with this issue. Consuming nuts like almonds and pecans have been known to bring down serum cholesterol focus inside the body framework. Nuts are additionally enthusiastically suggested for those people experiencing insulin obstruction issues like diabetics. Going to nuts rather than unhealthy food to subdue desires is likewise another better option. Containing fundamental unsaturated fats is likewise one more in addition to the moment that it comes to picking nuts as a better other option. Since nuts are sound and can be consumed in its crude structure, it is likewise one more added benefit to keeping these around and helpful as tidbits. Almonds are frequently used to standardize blood lipids due to their gradual process qualities, which help to keep the glucose levels reliably sound. Rich in a fluctuated measure of various supplements the almond is a well-known added substance to the flat eating regimen of most

Mediterranean individuals. The Brazil nut is additionally another nutritious nut which accompanies its own arrangement of advantages when consumed with some restraint. Noted for its omega 3 unsaturated fat substance, the Brazil nut is likewise a decent wellspring of calcium. Cashew nut is one more exceptionally famous nut that is many times consumed as a salted tidbit. Anyway, it would be a much better food item without the expansion of salt, as it is as of now a seriously delightful nut all alone. In certain regions of the planet these nuts are made into oils. The choice cycle ought to be finished with just enough information as relying entirely upon what the unaided eye sees isn't sufficient. For the most part lean meats from hamburger cuts ought to incorporate round, hurl, sirloin and tenderloin, while the cuts from pork or sheep would comprise tenderloin, flank hacks and leg. The least fatty pieces of the poultry would be the bosom region without the skin. However, there are many reasons individuals wipe out meat from their everyday eating regimen, there is no proof to show that this is a positive or negative decision nor would it be a good idea for it to be trailed by all. Anyway, the significant highlight here is the decision of the kinds of meats that would make the utilization sound and this would commonly mean meats with lesser measure of fat substance. However white meat is in no way, shape or form ailing in fat substance, it is by correlation substantially less in fat substance than red meats. The healthy benefit of consuming lean meats is very broad and adjusted. Lean meats have a for the most part higher and cleaner content of protein which is a vital contributing component to crucial primary and utilitarian advancement of each and every cell food and development. Lean meats are likewise a decent wellspring of fundamental amino acids especially sulfur amino acids. When contrasted with the stomach related rates the proteins in meats work quicker than the one contained in the beans and entire wheat range. Lean meat is likewise a decent wellspring of iron. Since lack of iron is moderate it is frequently not distinguished until a later stage where weakness has been created.

THE Advantages

Here is all the intention you'd expect to keep practicing good eating habits. We should promptly dive into the subject. Benefits You Get Better We could have an entire assortment of books about the wellbeing benefits of eating accurately nevertheless it wouldn't exactly cover what benefits really exist. The main benefit is that you gain control over your weight. By eating accurately, you similarly verify that your metabolic capabilities - most prominently your safe framework and your gastrointestinal framework - continue to work accurately. You're similarly safeguarded from grouped persistent sicknesses, right from cardiovascular illnesses like coronary conduit infection and hypertension to diabetes. More Savvy Practicing good eating habits implies you spend significantly less. Your bills at the grocery stores descend radically and you don't dive farther into charge card obligation assuming that is now an issue with you. Likewise, you save an immense pack on all the medical services costs you'd require on the off chance that any issue surfaces in view of your food gorging propensities. Less Poisons In Your Body A ton of food varieties these days are poisonous in light of the engineered synthetic compounds present in them. While you're endeavoring to eat accurately, you are significantly less prone to get these poisons into your body as one of the essential authoritative opinions of eating accurately is that you shouldn't eat anything that is man-made. Also, assuming you eat less, you'll similarly have the option to diminish on indecencies like smoking and liquor abuse. A glass of brew is practically inseparable from a night out with the young men. On the off chance that you eat less, you won't need the brew too. Likewise, you won't need that (at least one) obligatory smoke that you will more often than not have after every feast. More Actual Way of life When you eat better, you'll observe that you can take care of your responsibilities in a greatly improved manner. You can practice more, travel more, play more, work more and thus make your life more useful. That definitely beats being a fat good-for-nothing and relaxing around on the sofa the entire day, right? You can likewise be more engaged with your companions and friends and family and that definitely enhances your life. Great Public activity Disregard fat fetishism, people who are overweight don't look engaging. There are serious areas of strength for an untouchable weight on some unacceptable spots of the body. On the off chance that you're attempting to find an accomplice, your fat may in a real sense disrupt everything. Not just that, people who have no control over their dietary patterns and consequently their weight are peered downward on by society as being people who have no control over their fundamental desires. This kind of brain research exists, however not many people will talk about it. At the point when you eat accurately, you'll find that such issues vanish.

Wrapping Up

There are a ton of well-known eats less available these days, yet the greater part of them is unfortunate and at times even risky. This will make sense of how to eat a solid, adjusted diet forever and avoid undesirable weight control plans. Find out the number of calories your body expects to work consistently. This number might fluctuate fiercely, contingent upon your digestion and how truly dynamic you are. On the off chance that you're the kind of person who lays on ten hammers out plainly smelling a cut of pizza, then your consistently caloric intake should remain roughly 2000 calories for men, and 1500 calories for ladies. Your weight similarly has an impact in that: More calories are fitting for normally greater people, and less calories for humbler people. In the event that you're the kind of person who can eat without acquiring a pound, or you're truly dynamic, you could wish to build your everyday caloric intake by 1000-2000 calories, a piece less for ladies. Try not to fear greasy food varieties. You need to eat fat from food varieties for your body to accurately run. Yet, choosing the right kinds of fats: Most creature fats and a couple of vegetable oils are high in the kind of fats that raise your LDL cholesterol levels; the foul cholesterol is vital. Unique in relation to mainstream thinking, gobbling cholesterol doesn't definitely raise how much cholesterol in your body. Assuming that you give your body the right instruments, it will flush additional cholesterol from your body. Those apparatuses are monounsaturated unsaturated fats, which you should attempt to routinely consume. Food sources that are wealthy in monounsaturated unsaturated fats are olive oil, nuts, fish oil, and grouped seed oils. Eat a lot of the right carbs. You need to eat food sources high in carbs since they're your body's central wellspring of energy. Try to select the right carbs. Straightforward carbs like sugar and refined flour are immediately consumed by the body's gastrointestinal framework. This initiates a kind of carb over-burden, and your body discharges immense measures of insulin to fight the overburden. Not exclusively is the overabundance of insulin terrible on your heart, but it supports weight gain. Eat a lot of carbs, yet consume carbs that are gradually processed by the body, for example, entire grain flour, veggies, oats, and natural grains. Eat greater feasts almost immediately in the day. Your digestion decelerates close to the furthest limit of the night and is less productive at processing food sources. That implies a greater amount of the power put away in the food will be stacked away as fat and your body will not retain as numerous supplements from the feast. Have a go at eating a medium-sized feast for breakfast, a major dinner for lunch, and a little feast for supper. Even better, endeavor consuming 4-6 little feasts over the run of your day. Give yourself a cheat feast. Cheating doesn't mean pigging out on every one of some unacceptable food varieties one time each week; it infers partaking in a food you genuinely love one time per week. Two or three cuts of pizza on Sundays, or an immense cut of twofold chocolate cake on Saturdays. This cheat dinner will assist you with staying with the adjustment of diet, and in a couple of ways it's truly really great for your body. Unique events, similar to birthday celebrations in the family, consider cheat dinners. Get the propensity for eating gradually. It will fulfill you with less calories and will thwart indulging and corpulence with every one of its ramifications. Drink a lot of H2O. It causes you to feel more conscious and empowered, ponders your skin and causes you to feel fuller so you end up eating less! Chopping down pop and supplanting it with water will do ponder for you.

ABOUT THE AUTHOR

Isah Abdulwali Garba

Is an expert when it comes to food for a healthy life.
He is a final year student of Abubakar Tafawa Balewa University Bauchi (ATBU).
What makes this book unique is that everything inside is from personal experience.

Healthy Life Food

If you must leave a healthy life watch your intake

Isah Abdulwali Garba

Healthy Life Food

If you must leave a healthy life watch your intake

Isah Abdulwali Garba